# Growing Microgreens Step by Step Updated

## (From Seed to Table in 7 to 10 Days)

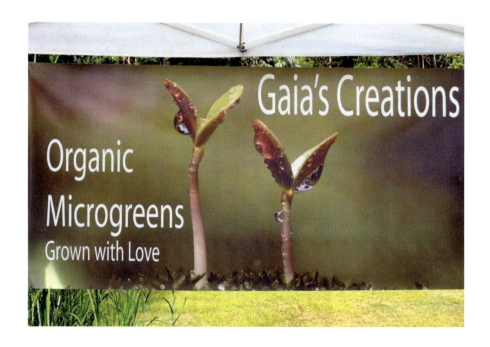

Susan Alima Friar

Updated First Edition

Text 2015 Susan C. Friar

Photographs Susan C. Friar

All rights reserved. No part of this book may be reproduced by any means whatsoever without written permission from the author, except brief portions quoted for the purpose of review.

Published by:
First Star Publishers
P.O. Box 1317
Paonia, CO 81428

Orders: GaiasCreations@live.com

Friar, Susan C.

Microgreens/Susan C. Friar – 1st. ed.

ISBN-13: 978-0-9910046-1-4
ISBN-10: 0091004612

## Dedication

To my microgreen students, supporters and friends:

Thank you for your encouragement, support and enthusiasm in our shared events.

To all the farmers of the precious seeds, thank you for growing these seeds with care for all of us!

And to my Dear husband, John, for your generous support of time, love and tasting as well as a lot of growing, harvesting etc.

# Contents

Foreword .................................................................................................. 5

Introduction ............................................................................................. 6

What Are Microgreens Anyway? ........................................................... 10

Why Grow Microgreens? ....................................................................... 13

Start with Success! ................................................................................ 17

Brassicas ................................................................................................ 26

Three Keys for All Micro Greens: ......................................................... 31

Shoot Peas and Black Oil Sunflower Seeds ......................................... 34

Beets or Cilantro ................................................................................... 40

Mucilaginous and No Soak Seeds ........................................................ 44

Different and Easy ................................................................................ 49

Harvesting and Storing Microgreens .................................................. 51

Quick Start Planting Guide .................................................................. 55

Troubleshooting ................................................................................... 57

Nutritional Information ....................................................................... 61

Recipes .................................................................................................. 63

Smoothies ............................................................................................. 63

Salads .................................................................................................... 68

Soups ..................................................................................................... 72

Entrees .................................................................................................. 76

Some Notes on Planting and Finding Peace with Mindfulness ......... 80

Resources .............................................................................................. 83

Mindful Inspiration and Reading ......................................................... 84

# Foreword

Susan Friar is dedicated to helping us all help ourselves to better nutrition, better sustainability, and better cuisine. Her well-illustrated and descriptive book Growing Microgreens is the definitive guide to producing excellent, delicious and sustainable nutrition for yourself and your family no matter whether you live on acreage or in a one bedroom bachelor's apartment. If you care about what goes into your body and what appears on your plate, this book is a must read. The techniques for growing your own microgreens are easy, fast, fun and fruitful. Research has shown the incredible amount of nutrients available in microgreens, and Susan has shown how we all can benefit from growing our own.

*Heartily endorsed by Jane Riley, M.S., B.A., Certified Nutritional Adviser.*

# Introduction

*"Peace is present right here and now, in ourselves and in everything we do and see. Every breath we take, every step we take, can be filled with peace, joy, and serenity. The question is whether or not we are in touch with it. We need only to be awake, alive in the present moment."* Thich Nhat Hanh

We live in changing times. I choose to change with the times, supporting the best I can for myself, my family and my community. It is my hope that you, the reader, will use what I offer to sample a new way to grow fresh greens while increasing your own food sustainability and improved health. In fewer than 10 days you can enjoy eating and sharing these colorful, fun smallest of edible plants. In the process you will also be supporting healthy agriculture and your greater community.

Actually, you have a much bigger opportunity in the minutes you spend tending your microgreen garden each day. In our busy lives we often attempt to do more than is realistic, many times ending up feeling stressed, tired, and overwhelmed. In encouraging you to grow your own microgreens I am offering you a challenge to take this opportunity to find some peace while nurturing yourself as no one else can. Curious? We'll learn more about this as we explore how to grow microgreens.

I began growing food in my 20's in the small village of Weston Vermont where my husband and I owned a small inn. Over my life I have had many teachers. Some of my best teachers were the staff at a non-profit organization, The Center for Land-

Based Learning, in Winters, CA. As a member of the staff, I facilitated hands-on learning programs with high school science students showing the impact of their choices and how they could help the environment through habitat restoration projects and various related experiences in agriculture, local government, wildlife management and similar community areas. Quite recently, this company has started training people to be farmers. I believe that we all need to be farmers on some level and care for the land and all the insects and critters which help our food and flowers and other plants to grow and thrive.

Some of us only have a windowsill or a patio on which to grow food. That is plenty of room for your microgreen garden. I began growing microgreens in my home in Taos, New Mexico where the soil was poor and I had so much light available. Sunflower and shoot pea microgreens thrived on my kitchen counter. From there I began growing other microgreens and continued to expand when we moved to Kauai where I sold and taught about microgreens. And now I still teach in Colorado.

Through trial and error, I grew greens in Taos, New Mexico and then in three different environments on the island of Kauai, having mixed results due to varying conditions. I also experimented with different soils and additions like earth worm castings, kelp etc.

I offer you an opportunity to create your own microgreen farm on your windowsill in your kitchen, on your porch or anywhere you have an appropriate environment. I promise that you can successfully grow a number of crops from seed to table in 7 to 10 days. This is fun, easy and a great way to teach young and old how to improve their health, create colorful salads, yummy soups, smoothies, stir fries and wraps or snacks.

As you read along, you will find mindful quotes that offer you a quiet moment in this new form of gardening. Choose one and allow it to open a window to a more peaceful possibility in your life.

So, let's get started! Here's a sample of one of my favorite microgreens:

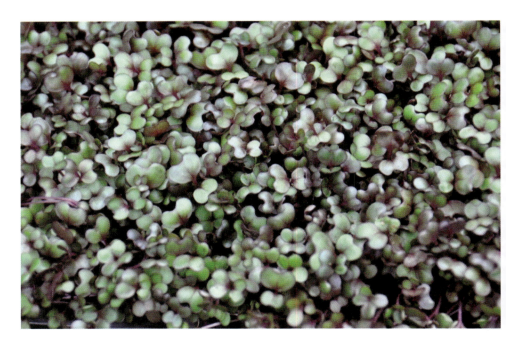

Red Cabbage

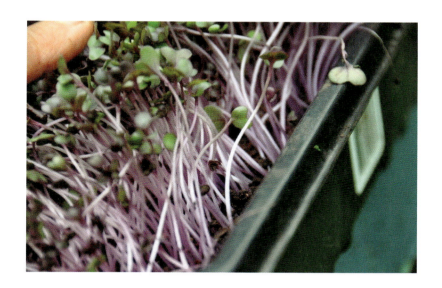

Red Cabbage has a mildly piquant flavor and glorious shades of green and lavender stems and leaves.

Hint: At this size purple kohlrabi has some of the same rich colors and flavor and is often less expensive.

> *"Gardening is how I relax. It's another form of creating and playing with colors."* Oscar de la Renta

# What Are Microgreens Anyway?

Microgreens first appeared in Southern California in the 1990's where they quickly gained popularity among fine chefs as a fresh and unique focus to highlight a particular dish. Soon these tiny plants were included in special salads or to complement a particular dish, such as with the intense cilantro/coriander flavor, delicate textures, color and interest.

They soon began showing up in Europe in the next decade. Many chefs have begun growing their own microgreens, knowing how important it is to have an herbal, floral or even hot and spicy green on hand to finish a particular presentation.

Microgreens are actually the smallest of cultivated green plants and are harvested at a young stage (1" to 2" in height) as opposed to sprouts which are germinated seeds. For microgreens, most seeds are planted dry (see chart), and germinate on healthy soil or a synthetic mat and are covered. Once uncovered, they can be in the light with good air circulation and moderate temperatures and humidity until harvest. Each is a complete plant which usually has a rich or intense flavor for its small size. In addition their nutritional value is becoming more and more of interest to health conscious consumers.

Microgreens are grown from vegetable, herb or edible flower seeds, and the whole plant is eaten. They are harvested just above the soil when the first two leaves (cotyledons) are fully developed and the actual "true leaves" (which appear in the middle of two fully developed cotyledons) may have started to form. In a moderate climate, to go from seed to table usually takes from 7 to 10 days. To the surprise of many, some microgreens are even more flavorful than the fully grown plants. This is especially true with cilantro and basil. **From bitter, to neutral to sweet**, microgreens are often given a separate section in seed catalogs to provide specifics on what to expect from these power packed greens.

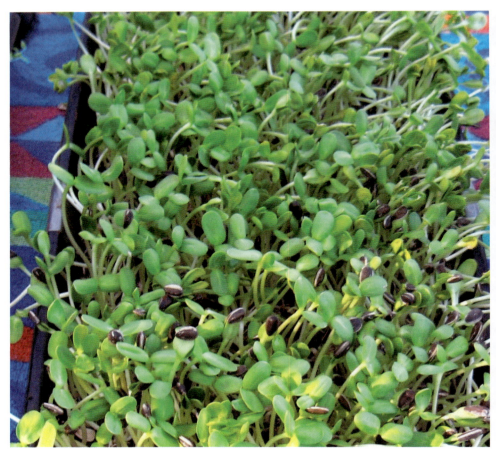

A bounty of "wild" sunflower microgreens in only seven days…………

# Why Grow Microgreens?

When beans, legumes, and seeds are sprouted, the enzyme inhibitors are neutralized. At this point, you have a germinated seed. By planting the seed, in an average of 7 to 14 days, you have a young plant with its first leaves that may have a higher nutritional content than the full grown plant and one that many find easier to digest.

Consider the following:

- You need very little space: a windowsill, a protected area of your porch or near a window in any room.
- You can have fresh, tasty and colorful greens year round!
- While sun light or indoor light is needed, indirect light from the sun on a cloudy day is often sufficient.
- You can grow microgreens in recycled containers or any pots with drainage holes: recycled clam shell containers, any plastic container or old flower pots.
- Amazing taste: Cilantro as a microgreen is incredibly rich. Delicate pea shoots taste like fresh peas from the garden 12 months a year! Some greens are stronger and some are milder than the full grown plant.
- The plants are fresh and ready to eat from your own efforts in an average of 7 to 10 days.

- Beauty in many forms: The rich color of red cabbage or beet microgreens adds a lovely contrast in delicate flavors and eye candy. Each microgreen offers a different taste and texture to your salad, wrap, sushi, and stir fry. Add as a garnish for your soup, entrée, dip or anywhere you would like a little flair.
- Increase your intake of vitamins, minerals and enzymes by incorporating microgreens in your smoothie (see recipes) or in a rich, pureed soup. In smoothies there are many ways to have a delicious, healthy combo without tasting of vegetables!
- Cost: Buying microgreens is expensive, and they are not as fresh. I will give you several seed company resources. You might even start a seed co-op with others to share in the shipping costs and to get larger quantities of seed for less.
- A mindful moment in your busy day: This is an easy way to begin a mindfulness practice, allowing yourself to breathe in the beauty of nature, connecting you with the earth and a moment of peace while spending a couple of minutes tending to your microgreens.
- A great project with kids or grandkids
- A wonderful gift for friends: When I began growing sunflower greens and pea shoots, I gifted friends with a small flower pot of partially grown microgreens. I also create starter kits of others.

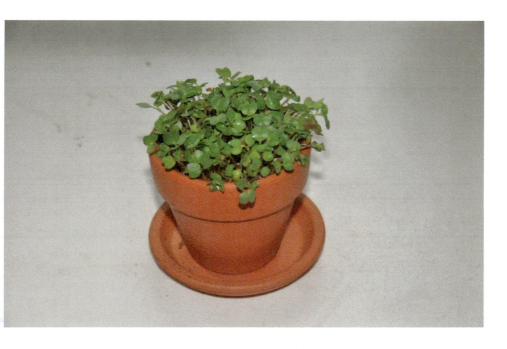

**Crimson Rose Radish**

Consider the power of the tiny radish seed which sprouts, roots and provides us with spicy greens in less than a week.

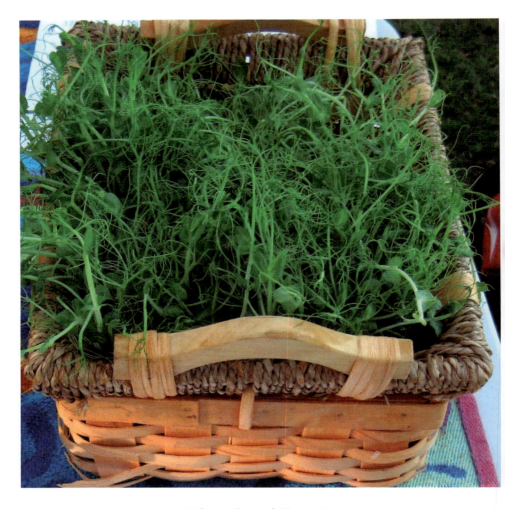

**A Gift Basket of Shoot Peas**

*"Everything that slows us down and forces patience, everything that sets us back into the slow circles of nature is a help. Gardening is an instrument of grace".*
*May Sarton*

# Start with Success!

Let's begin with my one of my favorite "no fail" microgreens...and I promise you once you see how pretty and easy these greens are, you will be ready to go. Can you believe that each week of the year, you can plant and harvest at least a half dozen plants and spend no more than five minutes a day (except when you clean trays...)

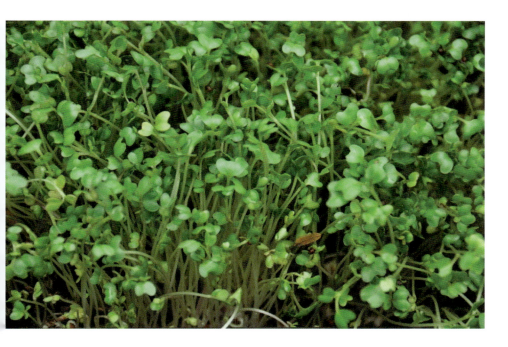

**Crimson Radish**

This little tray of radish took about 5 days in summer. Its cousins, broccoli, kale, cabbage and kohlrabi are just as easy.

I recommend that you purchase a few packets seeds which most appeal to you and some basic supplies. Note: The easiest microgreens to grow are brassicas and costs usually go down the more you purchase.

Here's what I suggest at this initial stage:

**First:** decide how much you want to grow at one time. Do you want to have enough for salad and possibly include micros in a smoothie several days a week? Or do you just want a little bit to see how much you like this new vegetable? And for how many people?

I estimate at least a cup of greens per day for one person which would mean either planting one "1020" tray a week (This measures about 10" x 20") or three of the smaller trays.

**Trays**: You can alternate a different green each week or grow two or three at a time. In the chart of greens, I will tell you how much seed you need to plant for a small tray or a "1020" tray. The small tray can be a plastic container with holes in the bottom to drain out water which you are recycling or you could buy ones like Greenhouse Megastore offers. There are three different sizes. This is the favorite and the small one on the seed chart.
http://www.greenhousemegastore.com/product/narow-seed-tray-black/flats-trays-inserts

There are three small trays which are inexpensive and sturdy. I have yet to find a sturdy "1020. Therefore, I always place one "1020" inside another so that they last longer. Plan on three trays per planting if using "1020": a doubled set in which to grow your greens and another tray inverted to act as a dome for your seedlings during the first 2-3 days after they are planted. You can buy them at any garden center.

**Alternatively** you can save your plastic "clamshell" containers with holes and tops from the store. Then you have a planter and a ready-made dome. Or use whatever you have with holes in the bottom.

**Use organic seeds**: Buy locally or check out the sources in the resource chapter, ½ to 1 lb. or more:

For certain seeds my favorite website is Tiensvold Farms, see Resources. (I love their sunflower, shoot peas, cabbage, corn, whole buckwheat, broccoli and other seeds)

For small amounts, I also have had good success with Todd's Seeds and Gourmet Seed. Get on their mailing lists…They offer deals and the latter offers free shipping from time to time. All have great quality seeds!

**Soil**: Some seeds are more demanding of nutrients even though they have enough inside to grow with very little help. Find a local source-- preferably one that has organic soil available. Experiment with organic potting soil, seed starter mix and soil and compost mixes to find one that you like.

**Compost** all you can to build fertile soil. And consider creating liquid gold ("worm tea") and worm castings by learning about vermiculture.

**Timing**: temperature (mid 60's to 80's), consistent air flow and consistent watering are your key factors. If you live in an arid part of the country, you may need to water more than twice a day. If you are in a wetter climate or with more humidity, you may water 1-2 times a day. In winter, plants will grow more slowly than the figures I have projected unless you live where your environment has an average of 70+ degree days and you have some sun regularly. Grow the hardier microgreens in winter: brassicas, tatsoi, sunflowers, and shoot peas.

**Fun**: Keep it fun and easy. Explore and discover one or two plants at a time. While I am not in your neighborhood, I am interested in your experience. Contact me if you would like to share or send pictures! I'll also include my blog address.

Once you have seeds, soil and trays, all you need is:

- One or two wide mouth pint or quart size canning jars with lids
- Plastic sprouting lids.
- Spray bottle and/or sprayer on your hose
- Scissors and unbleached paper towels or thin cotton cloth
- Press 'n Seal (optional) go to Amazon.com for description.
- Nontoxic liquid soap to clean trays (I use Dr. Bonner's liquid lavender)

- Small scrub brush
- Non-chlorinated clean water (with pH between 6 and 6.5) to use in trays with your seeds
- White vinegar

## Start Clean:

- Wash your sprouting jars and lids as well as cotton cloth you use on top of plantings.
- Before planting and then every time you harvest, clean out your tray and wash it in a non-toxic soap, scrubbing out any soil or root residue. Rinse well and dip it into a pan with white vinegar diluted in the water (one cup to one gallon of water).
- Wash your sprayer out regularly with soapy water or at least diluted white vinegar.
- Scrub plant residue off your scissors and wash them after each harvest.
- Also work with clean hands when planting or harvesting.

Now check out the chart on the next pages for the amount of seed needed, to soak seeds or not, and the time it takes from starting your seed to eating and enjoying your microgreens!

## MICROGREEN SEED VARIETIES FROM MY EXPERIENCE

| Seed | For Each Tray "1020" 5.31" x 14.57" Amount of SEED | Soak | Soaking Time | Germination Time | Seed to Table Note*** | Special Notes |
|---|---|---|---|---|---|---|
| Arugula | 1/4 cup 1-2 Tb. | no | n/a | 2 days | 5 to 8 days | Mucilaginous |
| Basil** | 1/4 cup. 2 tsp. | no | n/a | 4-5 days | 10-16 days ** | Mucilaginous |
| Beets* | 1/2 cup 3 Tb.* | no | n/a | 4 days | 6-9 days | *Scarify |
| Broccoli | 1/4 cup 1 Tb. | no | no | 2 days | 7 days | |
| Buckwheat | 1/2 cup 3 Tb. | yes | 6-8hrs. | 3 days | 7 days | |
| Cabbage | 1/4 cup 1 Tb. | no | no | 2-4 days | 7-9 days | |
| Cilantro * | 1/2 cup 2-3 Tb. | no | n/a | 7 days | 7-10 days | |
| Clover | 1/3 cup 2-3 Tb. | yes | 8 hours | 1-2 days | 7-9 days | |
| Corn | 1 cup 1/3 c. | yes | 12 hrs. | 1-2 days | 6 days | grows short |

* Scarify: scratch seed hull to speed up germination (further explai

NOTE: Lower or higher temperature and time in light will cause slower or faster growth

** Basil grows faster if placed on a heat mat

## MICROGREEN SEED VARIETIES FROM MY EXPERIENCE

| Seed | Amount of SEED 1020 Tray 5.31" x 14.57" Tray | | Soak | Soaking Time | Germination Time | Seed to Table | Special Notes |
|---|---|---|---|---|---|---|---|
| Cress | 1/4 cup | 1 Tb. | no | n/a | 3-4 days | 7-10 days | Mucilaginous |
| Kale | 1/4 cup | 1 Tb. | no | n/a | 1-2 days | 6-7 days | |
| Kohlrabi, purple | 1/4 cup | 1 Tb. | no | n/a | 2-3 days | 6-8 days | |
| Mizuna | 1/4 cup | 1 Tb. | no | n/a | 1-2 days | 7-10 days | Mucilaginous |
| Red Giant Mustard | 3-4 Tb. | 1 Tb. | no | n/a | 2-3 days | 7-10 days | |
| Radish | 1/4 cup | 1 Tb. | no | n/a | 1-2 days | 5 days | |
| Shoot Peas | 1 cup | 1/3 cup | yes | 8 hrs. | 1-2 days | 9-10 days | |
| Sunflower | 1 cup | 1/3 cup | yes | 8 hrs. | 1-2 days | 6-7 days | |
| Tatsoi | 1/4 cup | 1 Tb. | no | n/a | 2-3 days | 6 days | |

*"The moment one gives close attention to anything, even a blade of grass, it becomes a mysterious, awesome, indescribably magnificent world in itself."*
*- Henry Miller*

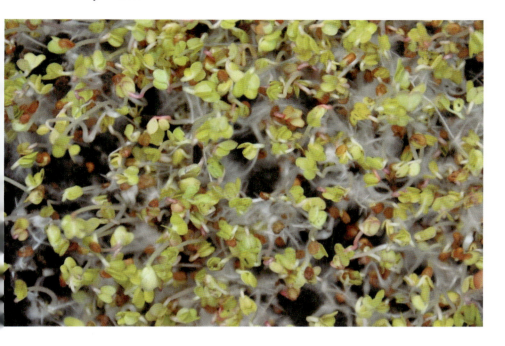

**Crimson Radish with fuzzy root hairs emerging**

Okay, so now that you know the basic necessities, let's go through the planting of three types of greens under which most vegetable microgreens fall.

Let us begin with the awesome brassica family, a true jewel of beauty and tops in nutrition and flavor from mild to spicy.

# Brassicas Update

Broccoli, kale, cabbage, radish, kohlrabi, many more

- Measure out enough seeds for your chosen tray.
- Fill your clean planting tray with organic potting soil or seed starting mix and loosen it well using your fingers; then dampen the soil thoroughly, but not enough to leave puddles. Make sure that the surface is <u>even</u> and at the same depth throughout the tray. It helps to press the bottom of another tray of the same size on top of the soil to even out the surface
- Lay the seeds on top of the soil, spreading them so that the seeds cover the whole tray. The seeds can cover the soil completely, but it is best for the growth if you don't have more than one layer of seeds. One eighth of an inch apart for small seeds is ideal, but don't try to place each one. Press the seeds lightly into the soil.
- Lay one thickness of paper towel, a thin cotton towel or a cut up cotton t-shirt on top of the seeds, covering all of the soil. Spray gently with a mist type sprayer (a bottle or your hose attachment) just until the towel or fabric is thoroughly damp.
- You have a choice to either cover the planted tray with an inverted tray (like a dome with holes) of the same or larger size or take one sheet of Press 'n Seal which is long enough to cover the top of the tray and secure it down with an inch overlap

on each end. It is sticky on one side. With the sticky side down, <u>make several slits</u> with scissors to allow some air flow through this plastic. Don't press down the sides so as to allow more air flow. Keep the seeds in the shade or covered with a dome (inverted tray) until they have rooted (for 2-3 days). Make sure they have good air flow.

- Place your tray on something waterproof (a baking pan or something with sides to catch extra water) and put it where there is some air circulation. NOTE: Seeds may develop fuzzy white around roots; these are **root hairs** and are a good sign. The key is consistency in water, some airflow and moderate temperature. You will need to spray the towel thoroughly whenever it dries out (once or twice a day).

- When you notice that the greens are pushing up the towel, uncover the greens. (in about 2-3 days). Do not re-cover them.

- Keep the soil moist as now it's the roots that need moisture consistently. Avoid overwatering or under watering. At this stage it is preferable to do bottom watering: place the tray in a sink (filled with one inch of water) for 15-20 seconds until you feel water seeping up through soil. At that time lift the tray and let water drain out. **Note:** it is usually best to water well once and then not water again until the soil is almost dry.

- Once uncovered, it should be 3-5 days until your greens are ready to harvest and eat. With all the brassica family you can cut just what you want each day while continuing to keep the soil moist. Just watch, you may get a second crop within a few days. **Note:** not all seeds germinate at the same time. So you may get a smaller, second crop.

## Time Summary:

- Plant and cover as directed until seedlings push up the paper towel 2-3 days. Keep towel moist.
- Uncover when seedlings push up cover and water from the bottom thereafter when soil almost dry.
- Harvest: (**do not water 12 hrs. before harvest**) cut in the morning (when cool) just above soil with clean, sharp scissors and shake off loose soil.
- Rinse and spin dry in lettuce drier. Lay out cut greens on a towel until dry. Layer gently and seal in a glass container.
- Greens, when dried, should last 5 days or more.
- Ways to enjoy: salad toppings, in your smoothie (with cinnamon & ginger…yum…see recipe on my blog: www.gaiascreations.com), pureed into a soup at the last minute and more.

**Note:** Putting a thin layer of soil on top of the seeds seems to result in a slightly different crop. So one time try growing the brassicas with just the thoroughly dampened paper towel on top and then

(Press 'n Seal) plastic wrap or cotton cloth or an inverted cover on top.

Another time lay out your seeds, and spread a thin layer of soil on top. Dampen soil well. Cover with a paper towel and dampen it and an inverted tray. Depending on your climate, your soil may dry out really fast and need to be watered twice a day or only once in the morning.

The paper towel or woven (not looped) cotton cloth are a quick way to see whether the soil and seeds are drying out.

You may not have to wash the greens. Just be sure to wash your hands and scissors before harvesting.

The paper towel method helps you to know when the soil is drying out. With paper towel or cotton toweling on top and no soil on top, your greens will be cleaner for harvesting.

**Note about cabbage:** Cabbage needs temperatures above 75 degrees F to germinate.

> *"Odd as I am sure it will appear to some, I can think of no better form of personal involvement in the cure of the environment than that of gardening. A person who is growing a garden, if he is growing it organically, is improving a piece of the world. He is producing something to eat, which makes him somewhat independent of the*

*grocery business, but he is also enlarging, for himself, the meaning of food and the pleasure of eating."*

— Wendell Berry, The Art of the Commonplace: The Agrarian Essays

# Three Keys for All Micro Greens:

1. Consistent watering (too much or too little can kill)
2. Moving air...if possible provide fresh air or at least a breeze through your window. If the plants are inside, try using a fan on low.
3. Once planted on the soil, Seeds need warmth to germinate in a somewhat low light environment and light to grow once rooted. On average once exposed to light, try for 10 hours sunlight and 6 hours darkness. Many will grow well though more slowly with less light.

**Note:** Don't worry about your water unless the plants are not doing well. Then test it. Ideal is pH 6 to 6.5 in water and without chlorine.

The following quote by Jim Rohn struck me as a great reminder:

"Take care of your body. It's the only place you have to live."

Now let's move on to the kids' favorites and my husband's too.

They are often like a wild child and are great to snack on or include in many dishes ...shoot peas and sunflower microgreens

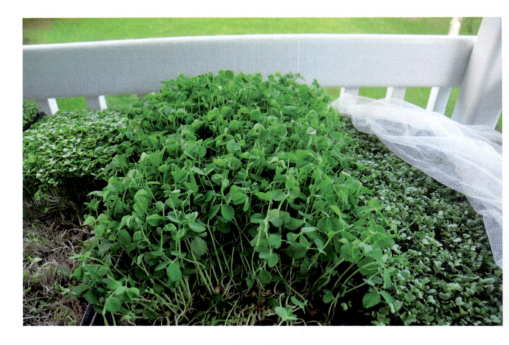

Shoot Peas

Pea shoots can grow repeatedly. Not just a one shot deal! They are a sometimes more tender when shorter. Added to the completion of a stir fry or whenever you want to add some visual interest or nutrition to a dish, they are a winner.

Here are some sunflower microgreens which are about ready to uncover:

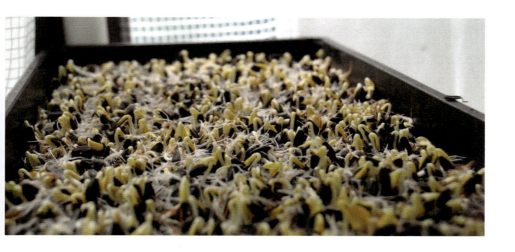

Read on to learn some of the differences in growing sunflower and shoot pea microgreens. And look forward to sharing some of these with family and all the kids in the neighborhood

# Shoot Peas and Black Oil Sunflower Seeds

1. Rinse well and soak seeds for 8 hours or overnight in a wide mouth canning jar with a sprouting top. Note: Peas can more than double in size. So plan accordingly for space expansion. Sunflower seeds will float. You need to fill sunflower jar full to the very top and cover with a canning top. Invert it while soaking as the sunflower seeds suck up the water and then some seeds may not get their fill.
2. After soaking, drain and then rinse seeds twice using a sprouting top so they drain well.
3. Set jars at an angle on dish drainer to drain fully.
4. Rinse them each morning and night until they have ¼ inch long tails (about two days). Invert the sprouting jar at an angle on your dish rack so the water drains out each time you rinse the seeds.
5. Lay the seeds on thoroughly dampened organic soil where you have broken up clumps of dirt and flattened the soil so the surface is even and same depth. Use another tray to flatten the dirt. (It is okay to have some sunflower seeds overlap.)
6. After "planting" sunflower or peas, mist and cover with another "planted" tray with holes. The weight of the upper tray helps the seeds to root and begin to push against as they reach up.

   **Notes:** Sunflowers are prone to mold if there is too much moisture in the air. Aim for good air flow to avoid mold and be sure to clean trays thoroughly between plantings.

Seeds may develop fuzzy white around roots; these are root hairs and are a good sign

7. The key is consistency in watering and good air flow. Water well on top or bottom-water and let dry out pretty well before watering again. .
8. Uncover the tray when most of your seedlings are lifting the upper tray(s) so that you can see them from the side with both trays in place.

   **Note:** Sunflower Greens need to be harvested before they develop a second or true leaf in the center of the first two leaves. The plant can get somewhat tough at that point.
9. Peas can be allowed to continue growing once you harvest them. Sometimes they will produce a second and somewhat fuller crop. Peas can grow up six inches or more and take about 10 days from soaking to harvest.
10. Cut just above the soil to harvest.

### Time Summary:

- Soak 8 hours to overnight. Then rinse well and allow to drain

- Sprout about 2-3 days till ¼ inch tails, rinsing twice a day.

- Plant until harvest 4-8 days

- Harvest: (**do not water 12 hrs. before**

**harvest**) cut just above soil with clean, sharp scissors and shake off loose soil.

- Storage: *rinse and spin dry in lettuce drier. Lay out cut greens on a towel until dry. Layer gently and seal in a glass container or re-sealable bag.
- When well dried, greens should last 5 days or more.
- Ways to enjoy: salad toppings, as a snack, added at the end of stir fries, in wraps.

  **\*Note**: You may not have to wash the greens until you eat them. Just be sure to wash your hands and scissors before harvesting. When storing in a plastic bag, poke a small hole as they (and buckwheat lettuce) like a little air. Greens don't like much moisture after harvest. Allow greens to dry in the shade after harvesting. Then layer greens with towel in your storage container.

*"Just look and just listen.*
*No more is needed".*
*~ Eckhart Tolle ~*

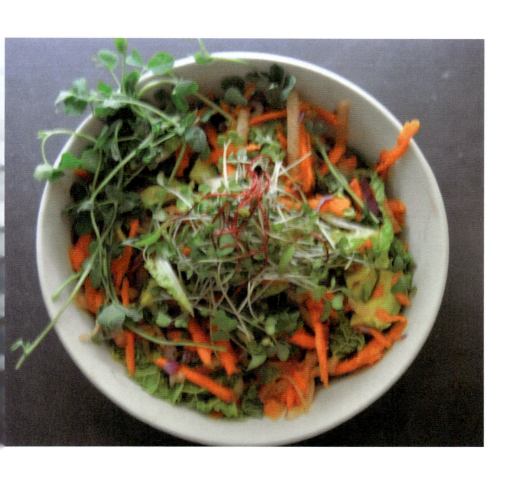

**Are you ready for lunch?**

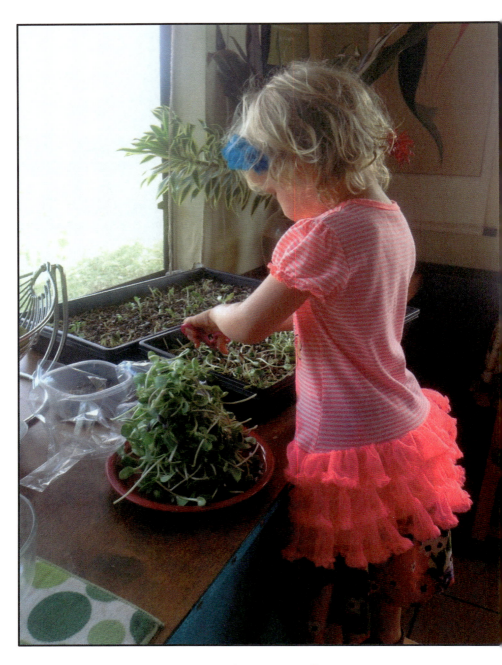

Mohala harvesting her favorite sunflower microgreens

When Mohala was three years old, we shared her home with her family. Upon being offered sunflower greens, Mohala would just stuff them into her mouth with pure pleasure. Now at four years of age, she is growing all kinds of plants, harvesting her favorite greens and feasting.

Now, catch your breath a moment and gaze into the rosy color of nature's bounty which offers beauty, a delightful sweet taste and lots of good nutrients in these beet microgreens.

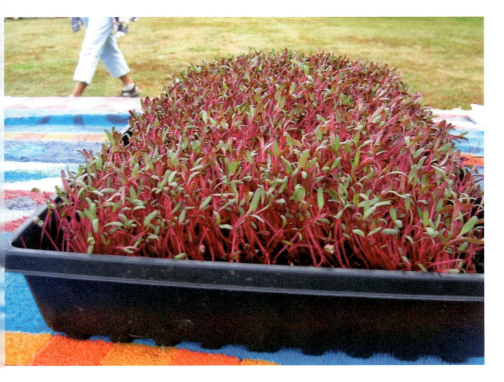

**Beets Microgreens**

*"Nature does not hurry, yet everything is accomplished"*
*~ Lao Tzu*

# Beets or Cilantro

1. These require scarifying to increase germination. Take dry seeds and put in a zip lock bag. Seal bag - removing air. With a rolling pin, carefully roll back and forth several times over the seed, firmly enough to break into the outer crust, but not go through crust fully. Listen for a crunch. You will not necessarily see any change visually.
2. Prepare a tray, filling it ¾ full with organic soil in which you have broken up any clumps of dirt and flattened so that the surface is even and at the same depth. Thoroughly dampen the soil.
3. "Broadcast" or spread the seeds as though you were planting a field. Press the seeds in lightly.
4. Cover the seeds completely with one thin layer of soil so that all the seeds are covered.
5. Mist soil well and cover with a paper towel or cotton cloth which you have thoroughly dampened. Note: Remember these seeds have not been soaked and will dry out more quickly.
6. Finally cover with either Press 'n Seal in which you put about 6 slits securing it on the ends only of each tray or cover the tray with an inverted tray with holes rather than Press 'n Seal. I think the latter allows more air flow. Note: I first cover most seeds with 1/8" soil as some stick to the paper towel otherwise.

7. When you notice that the greens are pushing up the towel, uncover them (about +/- 3 days). Do not re-cover them.

8. Keep the soil moist as now it's the roots that need moisture consistently. Avoid overwatering or under watering. Just water when the soil feels dry. Spray it and let the water drain out. As an alternative, place the tray in a sink (filled with one inch of water) for 15-30 seconds until you feel water seeping up through soil. At that time lift and let water drain out. Note: it is usually best to water well once and then not water again until the soil is almost dry.

9. Once uncovered, it should be 2-4 days until your greens are ready to harvest and eat. With cilantro, you can cut just what you want each day while continuing to keep the soil moist. Just watch, you may get a second crop within a few days.

**Note:** The beets or cilantro may take four to six days to begin to show above soil depending on your climate. Once uncovered, not all seeds may have germinated. I often put an inverted cover on top of the tray at night to encourage more seed germination. Also after first harvest, I cover cilantro for a day or two to get another harvest and remove the inverted top once I see a fair number of new plants. Always be sure to keep your growing greens' soil moist. I recommend that you water thoroughly once cover is off and allow the soil to almost dry out before watering again.

**Harvest Note:** Beets don't hold up well in the tray. It is best to harvest on the first or second day after they are ready. Cilantro lasts longer and often has the coriander seed still attached; this is a delicious treat for you to enjoy.

## Time Summary:

- Do not soak these seeds. Scarify before planting.
- Time from planting to harvest is 7-10 days, depending on seed and temperature. Keep moist as they were not soaked.
- Harvest: (**do not water 12 hrs. before harvest**) cut just above soil with clean, sharp scissors and shake off loose soil.
- Storage: rinse and spin in lettuce drier. Lay out cut greens on a towel until dry. Layer gently and seal in a glass container.
- When dried, cilantro greens should last 5 days or more. Beets may not last quite that long.
- Ways to enjoy: salad toppings, as a tasty and colorful garnish, as part of a special salad.

These cilantro Microgreens have a rich flavor that surpasses that of the full grown cilantro:

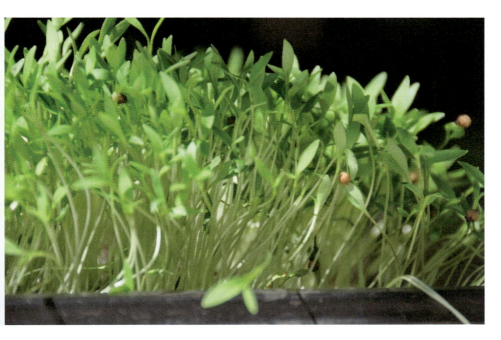

**Cilantro Microgreens**

*"The most precious gift we can offer others is our presence. When mindfulness embraces those we love, they will bloom like flowers."*

-Thich Nhat Hanh

# Mucilaginous and No Soak Seeds

This includes favorites like arugula, basil, mizuna, cress

1. **No Soaking**: Prepare a tray, filling it ¾ full with organic soil in which you have broken up any clumps of dirt and flattened so that the surface is even and at the same depth. Thoroughly dampen the soil.
2. "Broadcast" or spread the seeds as though you are planting a field. Press the seeds in the soil lightly.
3. Cover the soil completely with one thin layer more of soil so that seeds are all covered. Seeds may stick to towel. Adding a little soil on top will prevent this.
4. Mist soil well and cover with a paper towel or cotton cloth which you have thoroughly dampened. Note: Remember these seeds have not been soaked and will dry out more quickly.
5. Finally cover with either Press 'n Seal in which you put about 6 slits securing it on the ends only of each tray or cover the tray with an inverted tray with holes rather than press 'n seal. I think the latter allows more air flow. Just water when the paper towel is somewhat dry. Spray it well and recover with Press 'n Seal.
6. When you notice that the greens are pushing up the towel, uncover the greens. Do not recover them. Keep the soil moist as now it is the roots

that need moisture consistently. As an alternative, place the tray in a sink (filled with one inch of water) for 15-30 seconds until you feel water seeping up through the soil. At that time, lift and let water drain out. Note: it is usually best to water well once and then not water again until the soil is almost dry.

Once uncovered, it should be 2-4 days until your greens are ready to harvest and eat. With most of these, you can cut just what you want each day while continuing to keep the soil moist and just watch, you may get a second crop within a few days. **Note:** not all seeds germinate at the same time.

**NOTE: Basil** needs extra warmth. I recommend placing your planted tray on a **seed germination heat mat** and keep them covered until most have germinated. They will green up nicely after that. **Make sure they are misted and kept damp consistently.** This is one of the smaller and slower crops. So, **be patient. It may take a full two weeks to germinate and be ready to uncover.**

### Time Summary:

- Do not soak. In planting, be sure to keep them moist as they were not soaked.

- Time from planting until harvest is 5-10 days or more depending on seed and temperature (See chart)

- Harvest: (**do not water 12 hrs. before harvest**) cut just above soil with clean, sharp scissors
- Storage: *rinse and dry in lettuce drier. Lay out cut greens on a towel till dry. Layer gently and seal in a glass container.
- Greens should last 5 days or more when dried well.
- Ways to enjoy: pureed into a soup at the last minute, as garnish for certain dishes or with basil incorporated in an Italian dish and more.

**\*NOTE**: You may not have to wash these greens.

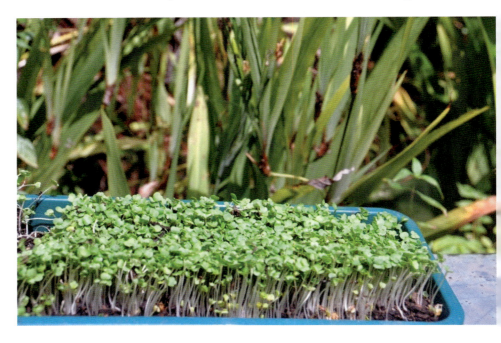

This small tray of tatsoi took 5 days to grow in the summer.

Next, let's try something different and fun...not what I expected. Check out these images.

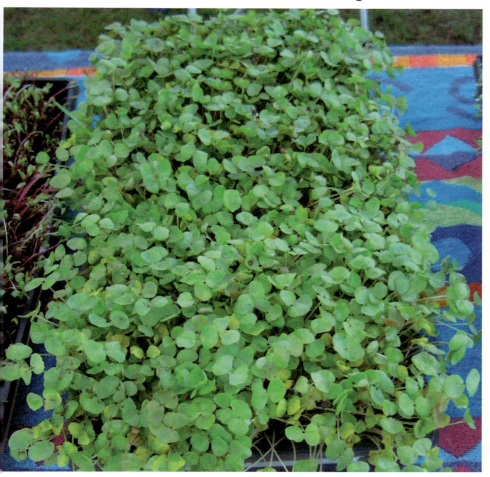

**Buckwheat Lettuce**


Buckwheat lettuce...buttery consistency and a mild flavor. Add nicely to any salad, smoothie, or as an unusual garnish with the buckwheat groats still attached. What is that, asks Aunt Iris?

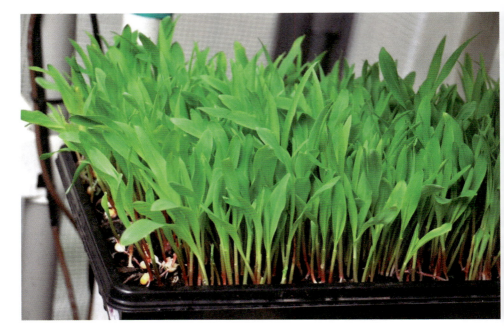

**Popcorn**

Popcorn, anyone? Yes really. It has a slightly bitter taste followed by a sweet finish.

# Different and Easy

- **Popcorn**: yes corn. You can soak it, but don't have to. If you soak, do so for about 6 hours and **plant it covering with soil as with brassicas.** It is a bit bitter followed by a sweet taste.

- **Buckwheat Lettuce:** Soak seeds overnight. Grow tails to ¼ inch and then plant like brassicas, and with the exception of a few groats left on top, there is nothing to remove. Groats may stick to the cloth so cover with a thin layer of soil and then a paper towel.

- **Clover**: most folks just sprout it or plant it as a cover crop. I get annoyed with removing the husks and find it easier to soak seeds **overnight** in a canning jar, rinsing well till they sprout a little and then plant. It grows nicely into small plants. If you have extra seed, put some in the garden to provide nitrogen to the soil! ** see picture on following pages.

**Grow all of the following as mucilaginous seeds** and **plant like the brassicas**. Remember **no soak for mucilaginous seeds.**

- **Tatsoi**: An easy to grow cool-weather plant, referred to as a Japanese spinach. Tatsoi has a gentle, slightly piquant flavor and can be picked over a week's time as long as you keep the soil moist and the plant appreciated.

- **Mizuna:** Flavor has a slight bite…so pretty and

easy. Try to grow some into bigger plants as well.

- **Cress:** A bit sharp in flavor...another pretty green.

## Time Summary:

- Soak or not as chart guides you. In planting, be sure to keep them moist, especially if they were not soaked.
- Time from planting until harvest is 5-10 days or more depending on seed and temperature (See chart)
- Harvest: (**do not water 12 hrs. before harvest**) cut just above soil with clean, sharp scissors
- Storage: Rinse and dry in lettuce drier. Lay out cut greens on a towel till dry. Layer gently and seal in a glass container.
- Greens should last 5 days or more when dried well.
- Ways to enjoy: pureed into a soup at the last minute, as garnish for certain dishes or with basil incorporated in an Italian dish and more.

*"While it may be difficult to change the world, it is always possible to change the way we look at it."*
*Matthieu Ricard*

# Harvesting and Storing Microgreens

- During the last 12 hours before harvesting, do not water the microgreens.

- Harvest when most microgreens are 1 ½ to 2 inches tall (or taller for peas and sunflowers).

- It is best to harvest in the morning or plants may wilt.

- Sunflowers are an exception. They need to be harvested before the 2nd or true leaves fill out. These will appear in the center of the first two leaves you see. You can harvest and eat most other microgreens as you desire allowing the cut area to fill in as more seeds germinate and grow up. When seeds are planted too closely, some will not be able to germinate for a second cutting.

- Cut the greens just a little above the soil with clean, sharp scissors. Lift up a section of the plants so that you can clip them just above the soil. Then shake off any loose soil and place them on a tray. If you cut more than you can eat, refrigerate the remainder.

- If the greens are very dirty, rinse them in your lettuce spinner, spin them and layer them in a dry paper towel. If they are not damp, I still layer them on a paper towel (to absorb moisture) and seal in a jar or container.

**Note:** I often don't wash my greens until I am ready to eat them as they take a while to dry thoroughly. None of them like to be stored when damp.

- If you are feeling overwhelmed, just grow the same crop a few times and get comfortable with that. I have given you a lot to start. It is simple once you do the process a few times.

> *"Just as you would not neglect seeds that you planted with hope that they will bear vegetables and fruits and flowers so you must attend to nourish the garden of your becoming."*
> — *Jean Houston*

## Harvesting Kale

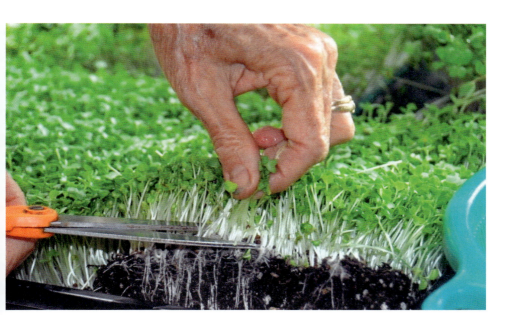

I gently lift the kale and the soil and cut it cleanly just above the soil.

Can you identify any of the microgreens on this page?

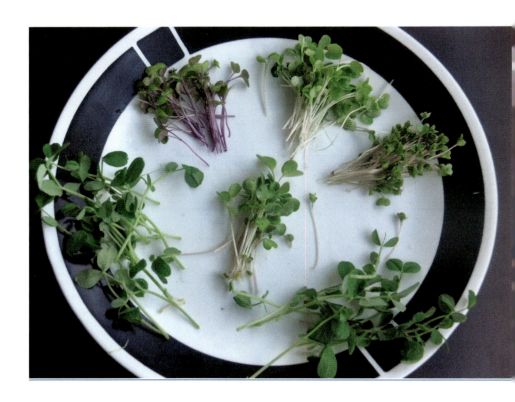

Start at bottom and go clockwise: pea, purple kohlrabi, mizuna, kale, and in the center, radish.

# Quick Start Planting Guide

- For peas, buckwheat and sunflower seeds: Soak the seeds for 8 hours in wide mouth quart size canning jars. Drain and rinse them twice and then drain them at an angle on dish drainer using sprouting lids.

- Rinse seeds morning and night and allow them to drain thoroughly until they have ¼ inch long tails.

- Planting -For brassicas: Fill tray with organic soil ¾ full and moisten soil thoroughly (no puddles once soil has settled). Flatten soil with another tray. Lay the seed on top, allowing them to completely cover the soil, but not on top of one another. Lightly press seeds down.

- With all brassicas, cover seeds with thin layer of soil. Then cover with paper towel and dampen well. Finally, put an inverted tray on top or Press 'n Seal to hold in some moisture. Only water when towel is dry. Keep in the shade or low light until they root.

- When seeds push up towel, uncover completely and let plants taking care they don't get too hot. Start harvesting when 1-2" high. Just harvest what you can eat. Mist soil a bit or bottom-water once a day or as needed until no more new seeds germinate (probably will have a smaller 2nd harvest)

- Planting-For sunflowers and shoot peas: plant one layer. After planting sunflower or peas, dampen well. Cover with another planted tray until the planted tray pushes the top tray up. Remove upper tray and keep in light watering from the bottom as needed.

- Sunflowers usually need more bright light during the rest of their growing. Only sunflowers need to be harvested before they develop a second or true leaf in the center of the first two leaves. The plant can get somewhat tough at that point.

- Mucilaginous Seeds: NO SOAKING...plant on damp soil and finish like brassicas (exception: cilantro and beets which you need to scarify first to open outer husk). Cover with soil and if desired, dampened paper towel until germinated. Be sure to keep moist until germinated. Cover with inverted tray or Press 'n Seal till greens lift the towel.

- Harvest early. After harvesting, allow greens to dry and refrigerate with layers of dry paper towel. Either wash and dry in lettuce spinner at harvest or just before eating. Some hold up better for 5-7 days if you withhold washing until just before eating.

- Wash trays with soap like Dr. Bonner's and then rinse with a diluted water and white vinegar mix. Let the trays dry out in the sun before next use if possible.

# Troubleshooting

- Start small. Plant small amounts. Get to know your seed varieties. Don't try to do everything at once. Buy just a packet of each seed until you find which flavors you particularly enjoy.

- Be sure to clean your trays thoroughly each time you plant a new crop. This will help you avoid disease and possible mold.

- If you do get mold or something else unwanted, you can pull out a little mold and see if that clears the problem. If not, it's best to start over. Clean your tray with non-toxic soap and a scrub brush. Then use a new sprayer and spray the tray with undiluted 3% food grade hydrogen peroxide. Allow the tray to soak in the hydrogen peroxide for 10 minutes while it kills the mold. Scrub the surfaces to make sure any residual mold is removed. Spray with fresh water and wipe the surface clean. Let the tray dry out fully before storing it or replanting it.

- Store the hydrogen peroxide spray bottle in a safe place and in darkness as it loses its effectiveness if left in the light.

- Plants need to struggle sometimes. Peas and Sunflower greens do best with a planted tray on top of the newly planted seeds until the sprouted greens have rooted, and the majority of the plants are reaching up for the sun against the upper tray. See notes for very humid climate.

- Yellow or somewhat pale crop, primarily with sunflower greens, may need more light and sooner. As soon as you uncover them, make sure they have enough sunlight so that they don't have to "reach for the sun" and then grow leggy to find sunlight. You can put them in the sun as long as it is not too hot or under a work light or LED light.

- If your plants do not thrive, test your water. Ideal pH is 6 to 6.5. Also, make sure that you do not have chlorine in your water. Seeds need to be from a recent crop. I try to buy what I can use in six months. I store them inside where it is relatively cool and keep them sealed.

**Note:** clay pots can pull water from the soil and so will dry out faster than other pots.

Plastic clam shells (fruit containers) have holes top and bottom) and are great natural trays with their own domes.

**Birds and other pests**: Birds love the sunflowers and sometimes want to nibble the peas. Below I have covered my trays with thin netting. Anything allowing light and air works.

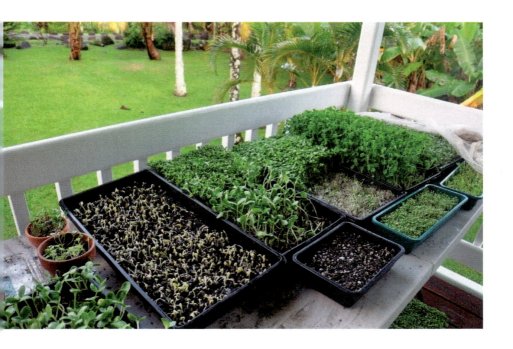

    Each time you rinse your seeds or check your growing greens or just think of them, know the gift you are for each other. By growing some of your own food, you help the farmers by buying their seeds and everyone who shares in the bounty. Breathe in the gift. Feel the love you give and receive in this process.

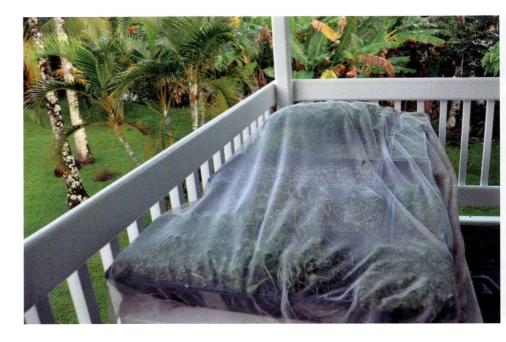

Mesh netting covering trays

This netting came from a thrift store. Anything will work which will let light through and keep the birds out.

# Nutritional Information

Some sources state that microgreens have more nutritional value than fully grown plants. I believe that they do though scientific studies have not fully verified this statement.

What is true:

- Microgreens contain a significantly higher percentage of phytonutrients and antioxidants. Most sites selling the organic seed state that these power packed greens contain a variety of nutrients, such as Vitamins A, B, C, E and K as well as calcium, iron, magnesium, phosphorus, potassium, zinc, carotene, chlorophyll, trace elements, amino acids and protein.

- According to the study referenced below from the University of Maryland and the USDA: microgreens contain a higher percentage of important phytonutrients and antioxidants and as much as 4 to 40 times more nutrients than the fully grown plants:
http://www.webmd.com/diet/news/20120831/tiny-microgreens-packed-nutrients

- While there are a number of articles such as those mentioned above, this is from the actual study:
http://www.ncbi.nlm.nih.gov/pubmed/22812633

- The following is from the Abstract: "Microgreens

(seedlings of edible vegetables and herbs) have gained popularity as a new culinary trend over the past few years. Although small in size, microgreens can provide surprisingly intense flavors, vivid colors, and crisp textures and can be served as an edible garnish or a new salad ingredient. However, no scientific data are currently available on the nutritional content of microgreens. The present study was conducted to determine the concentrations of ascorbic acid, carotenoids, phylloquinone, and tocopherols in 25 commercially available microgreens. Results showed that different microgreens provided extremely varying amounts of vitamins and carotenoids."

- Growing and being able to eat these greens soon after you harvest them has to be better than many options we have in our grocery stores, especially during winter.

# Recipes

While my suggestions are simple, hopefully, they will be a starting place for your eyes, taste buds and imagination. I rarely actually cook these delicate plants and so add them to my soups or stir fries at the end of the cooking as well as adding the microgreens to smoothies and salads. I only used organic seeds and preferably organic fruits and vegetables in these recipes.

## Smoothies

Each makes one large serving. I have found that the best machine for soups, salad dressings, smoothies, etc. is the Vitamix blender. Any good blender with a high speed motor will also work for most recipes.

### Summer Delight

- 1/2 cup of liquid, such hemp milk or other milk, coconut milk (try the frozen-it is great) or almond milk* (see recipe below)
- 1/2 cup of fresh berries or peaches or other fruit
- 10 almonds, soaked overnight and rinsed or 1 Tb. Almond butter
- 1/2 tsp. or more cinnamon
- 1/4 tsp. ground ginger
- 1/2 tsp. pure Vanilla extract

- 1 cup of microgreens (broccoli or other brassicas...radish if you want a little heat)
- 1 dash of Cayenne (optional)
- 1 banana, frozen or fresh

**Directions:** Make it to your taste. You can always freeze fruit and add it to chill your treat. Test to see what the balance is for you with ½ or 1 cup of greens. I find that with all the yummy flavors, I don't taste the greens much unless I add spicy microgreen or cilantro.

**Note:** addition 1-2Tb. cacao powder or your own super greens or favorite powdered shake mix.

## Super Food Drink

- 1 Mango or 2-3 ripe peaches or pears
- 1 Tb. Fresh, shredded ginger or 1/2 tsp. ground ginger
- 1 tsp. chia seed
- 1 banana
- 1 tsp. chlorella or spirulina or other super food
- Handful of microgreens and parsley
- 1 Tb. almond butter
- 1 cup hemp milk or other milk

**Directions:** Puree in strong blender. Adjust for desired consistency.

Optional: vanilla extract, cinnamon, nutmeg or ice cubes or frozen banana to thicken

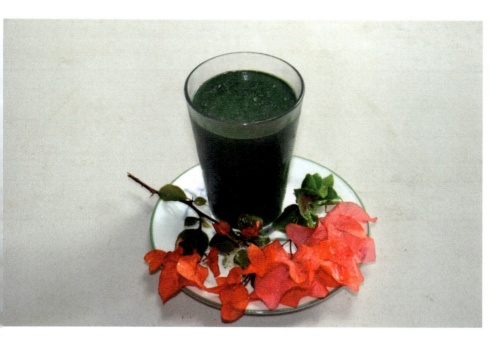

**Super Food Drink**

In winter, you might try one of these warming combinations to start your day or as a pick me up:

## Winter Chill Breaker

- 1 cup of almond milk (see the recipe at the end of this section to make your own) or other nut or seed milk
- 1/2 cup coconut milk

- 1/2 tsp. vanilla extract
- 1/4 to 1/2 tsp. each of ginger, nutmeg, and cinnamon or mix of cardamom and cinnamon
- 1 Tb. Cacao powder
- 1 Tb. Maca powder (optional "energy booster")

**Directions:** Blend together and if you want this a bit sweeter, add one pitted medjool date or 1 Tb. gentle sweetener, such as Stevia or honey. Blend again and place in a saucepan. Heat gently and **remove before it comes to a boil.**

**Note**: If you use Stevia, don't heat it.

## Chia Cheer

- 1 cup of almond milk (see the recipe at the end of this section to make your own) or other milk
- 3 Tb. chia seeds
- 1/2 tsp. pure vanilla extract
- 1/2 cup frozen blueberries
- 1 banana
- 1/2 cup of microgreens of your choice (broccoli, pea shoots etc.)

Optional: pinch of cayenne (it will warm you twice)

**Directions:** Puree all the ingredients in a blender or Vita Mix. Pour into a quart jar and allow the mixture to sit while it thickens for 15 minutes or more.

Eat as is or make this a topping for your oatmeal or quinoa or millet cereal.

To prepare millet or quinoa:

1. Heat 2/3 cup of water to boiling.
2. Add 1/3 cup of grain.
3. Let it come back to a boil and turn it to low.
4. Once the water is almost gone (10-15 minutes), turn off and let this sit until it soaks up the remaining water.

## Almond Milk

1. Soak one cup of organic almonds in one quart of water overnight.
2. Puree this combo in blender and press it through cheesecloth, nut milk bag or strainer. (Use nut puree in a pate or in some kind of nut loaf).

Yield will be about 2 cups of milk. Refrigerate and use within 4 days.

Note: You can dry the almond pulp in a 200 degree F oven or a dehydrator to use as almond meal in baking.

# Salads

## Rainbow Lentil Salad for 4

- 3/4 lb. green lentils
- 1/4 lb. pink lentils
- 1 small to medium diced red onion
- 1 diced sweet red pepper
- Arugula and cilantro microgreens
- 1/2 cup chopped walnuts
- salad greens

**Dressing**: (Blend well)

- 1/3 cup cold pressed, extra virgin olive oil
- 1/4 cup apple cider vinegar
- 1 Tb. maple syrup
- 1 Tb. Dijon mustard
- 1-2 tsp. salt
- 2 tsp. fresh ground pepper
- 1 tsp. ground cumin
- 1/2 tsp. turmeric
- 1/2 tsp. ground coriander
- 1/2 tsp. ground cardamom
- 1/4 tsp. freshly grated nutmeg

- 1/4 tsp. cinnamon
- 1/8 tsp. cayenne

**Directions:**

1. Rinse lentils well, drain. Place in a pot and cover with a 3-4 inches of water, bring to a boil, reduce to simmer. Check lentils for doneness after 15 minutes, but they should take about 20 minutes in total. You will know they are cooked if they still retain a slight tooth – al dente! Overcooking the lentils is the death of this dish. Be careful!
2. While the lentils are simmering, make the dressing by placing all ingredients in a jar with a tight fitting lid and shake vigorously to combine.
3. Finely dice red onion.
4. When the lentils are cooked, remove from heat, drain and place under cold running water to stop the cooking process.
5. Once cooled slightly but still a little warm, place lentils in a large serving bowl and toss with dressing. Add onion.
6. Let the flavors set for 15 minutes or so.

Just before serving, add desired microgreens. If using other options, such as greens, or cheese, add at this time.

**Optional:**
Shoot Peas, basil microgreens, soft goat cheese, and other vegetables

# Micro Cashew Coleslaw for 3-4

- 2 cups each grated green and red cabbage
- 1 cup carrot, peeled and grated
- 1/2 cup grated Daikon radish or 1 cup diced jicama
- 1 cup mixed microgreens: mix into salad (add radish microgreens) if spiciness desired; cilantro or basil for their rich herb flavor

Garnish: 1 cup of young shoot peas and ½ cup beet microgreens

## Dressing: Quick Version:

1. Juice 1 lemon and mash in avocado see photo on next page)
2. Mash soft creamy goat cheese into the cabbage and greens

- **OR** -

## Cashew Vinaigrette:

- 1 cup cashews, soaked overnight, rinsed and drained
- 1/2 cup water
- 3 Tb. cider vinegar
- 1 or more tsp. Dijon mustard

- 2 tsp. lemon juice
- 1 small clove minced garlic
- salt and pepper to taste
- 4 tsp. fresh dill, chopped or 1 Tb. dried

Puree dressing in blender and toss with salad. Let salad soak in dressing for 10 minutes. Garnish with beet microgreens and shoot pea microgreens.

**Optional:** Steam or gently boil whole beets till tender. Rinse and peel. Dice into bite size chunks. Toss with Dijon mustard, Spike, salt and Dill weed.

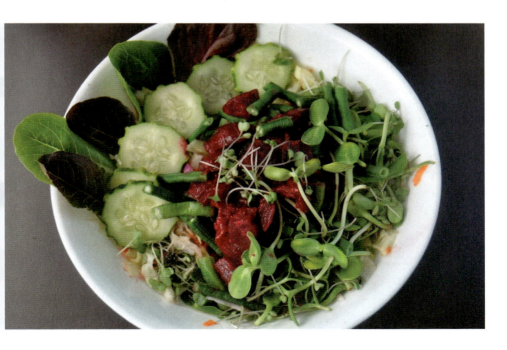

Dijon Beets with Lemon Avocado Slaw

# Soups

## Flex Soup for 4

- 2 Tb. Coconut oil (or olive)
- 1/2 to 1 large yellow onion, diced
- 1-2 tsp. ground cumin
- 1 tsp. ground coriander ½ tsp. curry powder
- 1 large peeled carrot, chopped
- 1 head of broccoli OR two zucchinis OR 1 cauliflower, separated into small florets
- One quart organic vegetable or chicken broth.
- One cup of greens you like (spinach, kale)
- Micro greens, 1/2 to 1 cup
- 1 tsp. Spike and salt and pepper to taste

**Directions:** Have fun and try any ingredients.

1. Sauté spices in oil with onion for a minute or two (Note: add Spike and salt at end of cooking)
2. While chopping other veggies, continue browning onion for a couple more minutes.
3. Add all vegetables except micros and green leaves. Stir in and add enough broth to thoroughly cover the vegetables. Simmer for 10 minutes until vegetables are softened. Throw in green leaves and let cook for one minute until they soften.

4. Put everything in blender with micro greens and a teaspoon or so of salt and 1/2 teaspoon of Spike. Puree. Serve & garnish with your choice of microgreens. You might leave some vegetables unblended for texture.

OPTIONS: add quinoa or brown rice or new potatoes or yams. Cook them separately.

(Quinoa: cook 1/2 cup in 1 cup + 2 Tb. Boiling water for about 20 minutes).

Brown rice: cook 1/2 cup rice in 1½ cups water for 30-40 minutes.)

Yam or sweet potato or white potato...if organic...scrub skin. Chop and throw in with vegetables to soup

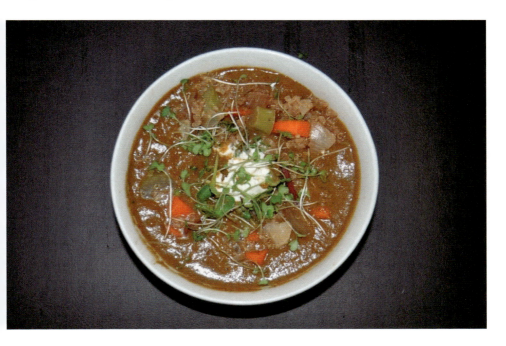

Flex Soup with Goat Cheese

# Moroccan Lentil Soup for 4

- 2 Tb. Coconut oil
- 2 tsp. garam masala
- 3 tsp. each of ground cumin and ground coriander
- 1 medium onion, diced
- 3 minced cloves of garlic
- 1 inch grated and peeled ginger root
- 1/8 tsp. fresh ground nutmeg
- 1 quart Water
- 12 oz. diced organic tomatoes
- 1/4 tsp. Asafoetida
- 2 diced carrots (1 ½ cup)
- 1 cup diced celery
- 1 tsp. sea salt
- 1/8 tsp. cayenne
- 1 piece of Kombu (seaweed)
- * 8 oz. cooked white beans
- * 8 oz. cooked garbanzo
- 4 oz. raw red lentils

* I used organic beans in cans that are BPA free. If you use dried beans, soak overnight. Drain, rinse and cook for about one hour in fresh water or until tender. Then add as above.

## Directions:

Sauté spices in coconut or olive oil for about one minute.

1. Add onion and cook for 5 minutes Then add Garlic and grated ginger root plus fresh ground nutmeg. Cook briefly- not allowing garlic to brown.  Add rest of ingredients.
2. Then grated ginger root plus fresh ground nutmeg. Cook briefly - and add rest of ingredients.
3.  Cook for 20 minutes until lentils, carrots, celery are cooked.
4. Allow to sit and let flavors blend for longer if possible.
5. Add cilantro or cilantro micro greens as a garnish and serve.

# Entrees

## Curried Vegetables for 4

- 1 small cauliflower, cut into florets
- 2 carrots, peeled & sliced
- 1 small winter squash or yam, peeled and cut into cubes
- 3 Tb olive oil or coconut oil, sea salt to taste
- Freshly ground black pepper, to taste
- 1-2 Tb. curry powder
- A pinch each of turmeric, cumin, cinnamon
- 1 Tb. tomato paste
- 3 cloves garlic, minced
- 1 small onion, diced
- 1/4 cup plain nonfat yogurt (or coconut milk or coconut cream)
- 1/2 cup fresh or frozen peas
- 1 tsp. grated fresh ginger
- 2 cups cooked organic brown or white basmati rice
- 2 cups tender shoot peas 1/4 cup cilantro microgreens

## Directions:

1. Place the cauliflower, carrots, and yams in roasting pan and coat well with 2 tablespoons of the olive oil.
2. Toss the vegetables with salt and pepper.
3. Place the pan in an oven preheated to 400 degrees. Roast the vegetables for 25 to 30 minutes, stirring once or twice.
4. Sauté spices in coconut oil. Add the onion followed by the garlic, being careful not to burn the garlic. Next add in the fresh ginger, and peas and simmer gently for five minutes. Add the pea shoots during the last minute and finally, combine this with the roasted vegetables and cooked rice.

Optional: Add some basil or basil microgreens as a garnish.

## Black Bean Tostadas for 4

### Ingredients

- 3 1/2 cups cooked black beans (2c. dried)
- 1 medium onion, diced
- 2-3 cloves garlic, minced
- 1 Tb. ground cumin
- 1 Tb. ground coriander
- 1½ tsp. ground chili powder
- 1-2 tsp. dried basil

- 1 tsp. Spike seasoning
- 1/2 tsp. salt
- Fresh ground pepper
- 3-4 Tb. Organic tomato paste
- Coconut oil
- 2 cups diced organic vegetables (i.e. broccoli, zucchini, chayote, peppers, etc.)
- 8 organic sprouted corn tortillas
- 1-2 cups microgreens (especially pea)

Optional: Creamy goat cheese or cashew cheese

## Directions

1. Soak beans overnight. Rinse and with fresh water, simmer until tender (1-2 hours).
2. Sauté onion in coconut oil adding spices * within the first minute.
3. When onion is browning, add garlic for a minute or so.
4. Add 2 cups of vegetables and the rest of seasonings and sauté for a couple of minutes.
5. Then add the cooked beans. Mash in the beans and add the tomato paste and cook a few minutes more till flavors mix while vegetables are still a bit al dente. Check for seasoning.
6. Sauté each tortilla in a little (1 Tb.) coconut oil turning once.

7. Place the tortilla folded in half on a plate and hold in warming oven until all tortillas are warmed.

8. Fill tortillas with bean-vegetable mix and a little goat cheese, or cashew cheese if desired. Put a quarter cup of microgreens inside the tortilla and enjoy.

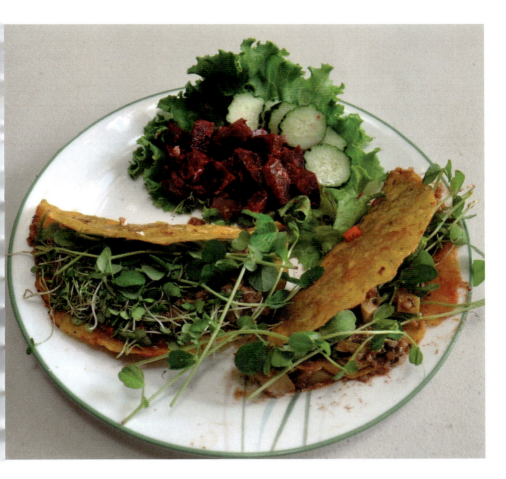

**Black Bean Tostadas & Dijon Beet Salad**

# Some Notes on Planting and Finding Peace with Mindfulness

We are all energy and are surrounded by energy in many forms. In our busy lives, we often are so preoccupied that we lose touch with ourselves, who we are, and what our bodies are experiencing as well as much of what surrounds us in our experience.

Each living plant, human, animal, insect, is first and foremost energy. If we were to look inside, we would see molecules constantly moving. At the same time, there are so many processes of which we are not even aware.

I think of water and air as the energy highway carrying our thoughts, our feelings, and our perceptions of our inner and outer world. When we care for plants, other people, or ourselves, our energy or vibration speaks more than our words. Have you ever walked into a room and felt tension or anger present in someone else? Plants sense what we carry: fear, sadness, anxiety. Plants feel our energy. (See Resources Dr.Marsaru Emoto)

As with humans, plants hold a lot of water and will react to our vibration, our thoughts and the energy we hold while working with them.

Some plants responded to my anxiety before market day. The sunflowers actually were less productive on those days. When I didn't worry, the plants knew it.

As I began to learn that I was part of the cause of some ill health, I began reading about mindfulness. The simplicity of Thich Nhat Hanh's words resonated very deeply. Congressman Tim Ryan's book: *A Mindful Nation,* brought home how out of touch I was with my body and my emotions. I began a daily practice which helped me connect to both my emotional and physical states, and to understand myself better and how I could change my response to "stress" in 10-20 minutes daily.

I just mention these resources and experience as tools you can explore. They have helped me have a more peaceful life, to let go of what no longer serves me, and to be truly present each day?

During at least the past century, we have progressed so much while also losing touch with ourselves and nature at times  This **stress** manifests in our emotions and in our body in many forms and causes imbalances as we cope with our lives in a variety of  ways.

If you would like to relieve some stress and tension, there are several ways to begin. Throughout this book, you found quotes from some wise people who share their lessons in releasing what does not serve them and being in the present. You might take one quote a day or pin one up where you will see it (above the kitchen sink or above the bathroom mirror) to remind you to breathe, to be present and allow yourself a moment to connect with your body, the world around you, the gift of today.

Also while you are working with these vibrant microgreen seeds, allow yourself to be truly present, to focus on the present experience, feeling the soil, the seeds, noticing how you feel as you work with this vibrant life force. Gift yourself in whatever way this experience speaks to you.

We are often taught to give, to support, to work hard and to succeed. Without self-care, and taking time to be present, eventually, we burn out, and our essence says, enough. What about me! How can we be present and support others if we don't honor ourselves?

Thank you for taking the time to learn about microgreens. I hope you will share whatever you learn with your family and friends. Have fun!

*"Life is a flowing stream, forever passing away and as constantly being renewed. The energy that brings us life is supplied from many different sources, most of them, beyond our vision of experience."*

*(The Web of Life p. 14)*

# Resources

**Seeds:**

- For small amounts up to one pound: www.toddsseeds.com
- For one pound or more, Tiensvold Farm in Nebraska at: http://shop.eatorganicbuffalo.com/Certified-Organic-seed_c2.htm
- For some unusual seeds: www.gourmetseed.com

Gourmet Seed is located in New Mexico and many of their seeds come from Italy.

Get on Todd's and Gourmet Seeds' mailing lists for special money saving opportunities.

**Websites:**

www.growingmicrogreens.com

www.sproutpeople.org

www.greenhousemegastore.com

# Mindful Inspiration and Reading

*A Mindful Nation* by Congressman Tim Ryan

*Peace Is Every Step* by Thich Nhat Hanh

*Inside-Out Healing* by Richard Moss

*The True Power Of Water* by Masaru Emoto


**Contacting Susan Alima Friar:**

If you would like to share your experiences or challenges and photos, feel free to contact me at gaiascreations@live.com

I do offer some coaching support.

Check out my blog: www.gaiascreations.com

And/or my Facebook page: www.facebook.com/gaiascreationscom


> *"In the end, just three things matter:*
> *How well we have lived*
> *How well we have loved*
> *How well we have learned to let go"*
> *— Jack Kornfield*

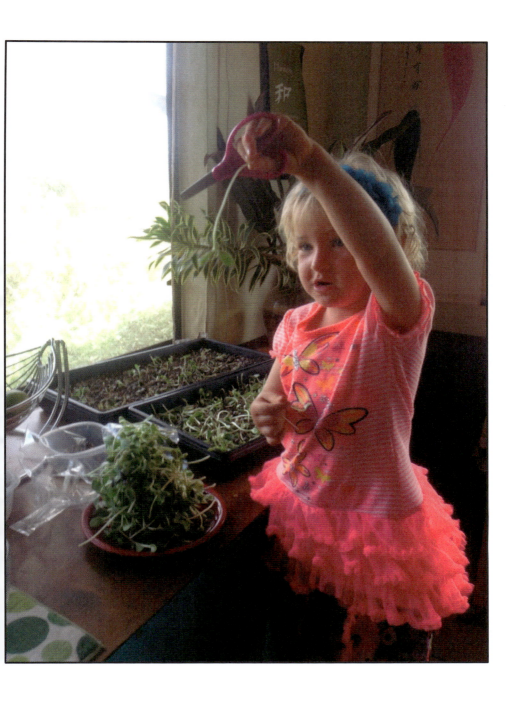

Happy Harvester

Made in the USA
Charleston, SC
24 September 2016